Affordable Paleo Cooking

Healthy and Budget-Friendly Paleo Meals

Contents

About This Book

This book is a compact cookbook that offers you the tools you need to cook healthy, Paleo friendly and budget-friendly meals. Paleo dieting is a new trend that has taken over the world, and is quickly becoming a lifestyle for many people. Each recipe in this book is highly affordable, and will give you the benefits of eating a Paleo diet while keeping the flavors fresh and delicious. The book starts out with soups and stews, continues to delicious main dishes, then the must-have side dishes and then delicious desserts. Cook all these recipes at home while saving a few extra dollars.

Introduction

Paleo dieting is simple. All you have to remember when looking at food is the question: "Could a caveman eat this?" If the answer is yes, then the food product is 100% Paleo. Basically, Paleo dieters occupy the school of thought that food is best in its simplest and most natural form. Therefore, any processed food is out. This includes processed sugars, grains and even processed fruits and veggies. Due to the lack of processed foods in the Paleo diet, this diet is extraordinarily healthy.

Paleo followers often have lower body mass indexes, better cardiovascular health, lower blood pressure, and a lower incidence of most diseases, even including the common cold. Plus, the best part about following the Paleo lifestyle, is that unlike other dieting lifestyles (i.e. vegetarianism and veganism) Paleo followers do eat meat. Therefore, this lifestyle is often easier for most people to follow and stick with than other healthy-eating lifestyles. Whether you are new to the Paleo lifestyle or you are a seasoned veteran, this Paleo cookbook will be a great resource for fresh and delicious meals that you and your family and friends will adore. Plus, all of the recipes in this cookbook are affordable, especially if you shop for your fruits and veggies locally.

Soups and Stews

Vegetable Rice Soup

Servings 4
1 ½ C. Brown Rice, uncooked
1/4 lb. Mushrooms, sliced
2 Carrots, peeled and sliced
1/2 White Onion, diced
2 Celery Stalk, sliced
1 cup Red or Green Pepper, diced
2 Large Red Potatoes, diced
2 cups Broccoli, chopped
2 1/2 Vegetable bouillon cubes
2 Cloves garlic, minced
1 tbsp. Black pepper
5 C. Water

Place all ingredients in a large stockpot, except the brown rice. After the broth has boiled, add the brown rice and cover the soup. Simmer for 20 minutes, and serve piping hot.

Pot Roast Soup

Servings 4
1 ¼ lb of Stew Meat
1 White Onion, diced finely
3 Large Carrots, peeled and diced
1 cup of Butter Nut Squash, diced
1 Large Tomato, diced
½ lb of Button Mushrooms, diced
2 cups of Broth (Vegetable, Chicken or Beef)
1 tbsp. Black Pepper
½ tbsp. Salt
1 Large pinch Oregano
1 Large pinch Basil

Throw all of your vegetables and your diced stew meat into your crock pot. Next, add the broth of your choice, and all of your spices. Cover, and cook on high for 5-6 hours, or until your stew meat and vegetables are cooked through thoroughly.

Spinach Tomato Soup

Servings 4
1 Medium Onion, diced finely
1 ½ bags of Baby Spinach
2 Large Fresh Red Peppers, diced
2 Large Fresh Tomatoes, diced
2 Large Fresh Tomatoes, peeled and crushed
4 cloves of Garlic, minced
1 tsp. Basil
1 tsp. Oregano
4 cups Chicken Broth
Juice from 1 Lemon
2 tsp. Black Pepper
1 tsp. Salt
Coconut Oil for cooking (or Olive Oil)

Place your coconut/olive oil in a saucepan and add your onions. Sweat the onions for about 5 minutes, and then add your peppers, spinach, diced and crushed tomato and your spices. Cook uncovered over medium heat for a few minutes while stirring the soup. Next, add in the chicken broth and simmer, covered for 30 minutes. Before you serve your soup, squeeze the juice of one lemon into the pot, stir, and then add more salt and pepper to taste.

Black Bean Soup

Servings 4
3 cups Black beans, soaked overnight
4 cups Water
3 cups Vegetable Broth
1 Yellow Pepper, diced finely
1 Jalapeno, chopped and deseeded
1 Celery stalk, chopped finely
1 Medium White Onion, diced
2 Cloves garlic, minced
Salt and Pepper to taste
Cilantro

Add all of your ingredients, except your cilantro, into a large stockpot. Cook on medium high until the soup boils, and then cover it and simmer for 30 minutes. When ready to serve, roughly tear your cilantro and garnish each bowl with a few pieces.

Potato and Leek Soup

Servings 4
1 Package of Bacon
2 White Sweet Potatoes
4 Medium Carrots, peeled and diced
5 Stalks of Celery, chopped
1 Medium Onion, diced finely
3 Leeks, washed and diced
3 Sprigs of Green Onion, diced
4 cups Vegetable Stock (or Chicken)
Salt and Pepper to Taste
Olive oil

First grab a sauté pan and begin cooking your bacon. Once it is finished cooking, lay your bacon on a wire rack, or on a plate covered in paper towels to drain the grease from it. Next, throw your celery, carrots, and white onion into a saucepan with olive oil to sweat them out. After they have cooked for a few minutes, add your sweet potatoes, leeks, green onion and your broth (vegetable or chicken) to the pot. If your broth isn't covering all of your vegetables yet, then add water to your stockpot until your veggies are covered. Cook on medium-high heat until all of your potatoes and leeks are cooked through. Next, use an immersion blender (or a regular blender) to blend all of your ingredients together. Blend until smooth and then add salt and pepper to taste. Serve piping hot, with a sprinkle of bacon on top.

Roasted Cauliflower Soup

Servings 4
1 Head of Cauliflower, diced
2 cloves of Garlic, minced
1 tbsp. Olive Oil/Coconut Oil
4 cups Vegetable Broth
1 cup Broccoli, diced
½ cup White Onion, diced
2 cups Milk
Pepper to taste

Place your cauliflower and broccoli onto a baking sheet and lightly sprinkle with pepper and olive oil. Place the baking sheet in the oven at 350 degrees Fahrenheit for 10 minutes. Next, place your cauliflower, broccoli, onion, garlic and vegetable broth into a stockpot. Boil, and allow to cook for 10 minutes to cook the vegetables all of the way through. Add your milk and more pepper (if needed), then blend with an immersion blender until smooth. Serve hot with a sprinkle of cheese, bacon, or green onion.

Main Dishes

Mushroom Salad Cups

Servings 4
4 Portobello Mushrooms, cleaned
Olive Oil
2 cloves Garlic, minced
Salt and Pepper
1 Head Romaine Lettuce, washed and chopped
½ Lemon, juiced
¼ cup Balsamic Vinegar

Preheat your oven to 350 degrees Fahrenheit. Clean and de-stem your mushrooms, then drizzle them with olive oil and liberally sprinkle salt and pepper over the mushroom caps. Sprinkle the minced garlic over the mushrooms and then place them in the oven for 30 minutes. Remove the mushroom caps, and drain any excess water from them. Next, grab the lettuce and dress it with balsamic vinegar and olive oil. Add salt, pepper and lemon juice to lettuce and stir. Top each mushroom cap with lettuce and sprinkle cheese on top if you desire.

Rice and Veggie Bowl

Servings 4
2 cups Brown Rice, uncooked
1 Red Pepper, diced
1 Yellow Pepper, diced
1 Medium Onion, diced
2 large Carrots, peeled and diced
½ Head of Broccoli, chopped
4 cloves Garlic, minced
1 cup Vegetable Broth
4 cups of Water
Olive Oil
Salt and Pepper

Place your vegetable broth and water into a saucepan and bring it to a boil. Next, add your rice, and simmer, covered for twenty minutes, or until the rice is fluffy and cooked. Sweat your onion in a medium sauté pan for 2-3 minutes with olive oil. Add the rest of your vegetables and garlic and sauté until the vegetables are cooked through, but still crunchy. Serve 1 cup of rice with sautéed veggies on top and add salt and pepper to taste.

Zucchini Lasagna

Servings 4
3 Medium Zucchini, sliced thinly
1 lbs Grass Fed Beef
1 bag Baby Spinach
1 Medium White Onion, diced
1 Large Tomato, diced
1 Can Tomato Paste
5 cloves Garlic, minced
2 tbsp. Basil
2 tbsp. Oregano
½ tsp. Salt
1 tsp. Pepper
Olive Oil

Sweat the garlic and onion in a large stockpot for 3 minutes in olive oil. Add your ground beef and brown. Next, add the tomatoes, tomato paste, basil, oregano, salt, and pepper to the mixture and cook for 10 minutes. Then add the spinach and cook until wilted. Then, layer your zucchini slices in a baking pan. On top of your zucchini place a layer of the meat mixture, and then add more zucchini. Continue layering until you run out of ingredients. Next, bake the lasagna covered in foil for 30 minutes in a 350 degrees Fahrenheit oven.

Vegetable Scrambled Eggs

Servings 4
8 large Eggs
1 cup of Asparagus, chopped
½ cup Tomato, diced
¼ cup Onion, dice
1 cup Broccoli, chopped
Salt and Pepper to Taste
Olive Oil

Sautee your vegetables in olive oil in a sauté pan over medium heat. Meanwhile, mix your eggs together with salt and pepper. Then, add your veggies to your egg mixture and put it all back in the oiled sauté pan. Cook until your eggs are scrambled, stirring frequently.

Stuffed Mushrooms

Servings 4
4 Large Portobello Mushrooms, cleaned and stems removed
1 lb Grass Fed Beef
3 stalks Celery, diced
1 White Onion, diced
½ Red Pepper, diced
4 Mushroom Stems, chopped
5 cloves Garlic, minced
2 tbsp. Oregano
½ tsp. Paprika
Salt and Pepper
Olive Oil

Preheat your oven to 400 degrees Fahrenheit, and then clean your mushrooms with a damp paper towel. Place your cleaned mushrooms on a baking sheet. Next, brown your ground beef and then add all of your veggies, garlic and mushroom stems to the meat. Cook until the veggies are softened. Next, scoop the mixture into the mushroom caps and tent your baking sheet with foil. Bake for 25 minutes.

Bacon Stuffed Mushrooms

Servings 4
4 Large Portobello Mushrooms, cleaned and stems
removed
1 lb. Bacon, diced
½ White Onion, diced
½ Green Pepper, diced
1 Medium Tomato, diced
4 Mushroom Stems, diced
3 Cloves Garlic, minced
1 Bag Baby Spinach, chopped

Preheat your oven to 400 degrees Fahrenheit, and clean
and de-stem your mushrooms. Next, cook your bacon and
dice it up once it is cooked. Add your bacon, white onion,
garlic, green pepper, tomato, and mushroom stems back
into your sauté pan and cook until the veggies are soft.
Next, add in your spinach and cook until the spinach is
wilted. Scoop your mixture into your mushrooms and bake
for 20 minutes.

Vegetable Stir-fry

Servings 4
2 cups Broccoli, chopped
1 Red Pepper, diced
1 Yellow Pepper, diced
1 cup Button Mushrooms, sliced
1 Large Carrot, peeled and diced
1 cup Fresh Pineapple, diced
1 cup Cabbage, diced
1/8 cup Tamari Sauce
2 cups Cooked Brown Rice
4 eggs, scrambled
Salt and Pepper to Taste
Olive Oil

Place all of the vegetables and mushrooms into a sauté pan with a bit of Olive oil and sauté until the veggies are cooked through. Add a splash of tamari sauce for flavoring then add your cooked rice. Cook for 5-10 minutes in the sauté pan and then serve with scrambled eggs on top.

Asparagus, Broccoli and Egg Casserole

Servings 4
12 Eggs
2 Medium Onions, diced
1 Bunch Asparagus, diced
1 Head Broccoli, chopped
3 cloves Garlic, minced
Salt and Pepper
Olive Oil

Beat your eggs with salt and pepper and set aside. Next, place your asparagus, broccoli and garlic into a sauté pan and heat over medium heat. Cook for 10 minutes with olive oil as needed. Add your veggies to your beaten eggs and then pour the mixture into a baking dish. Bake in a 350 degree Fahrenheit oven for 40 minutes.

Paleo Tacos

Servings 4
1 lb. Grass Fed Ground Beef
½ tbsp. Cumin
½ tbsp. Garlic Powder
1 tsp. Black Pepper
1 cup Red Pepper
1 cup Yellow Pepper
1 Medium Tomato, diced
1 tbsp. Chili Powder
Pinch of Salt
Romaine Lettuce

Brown your beef with the cumin, garlic powder, chili powder and salt. Then add your peppers and tomato. Cook until the peppers and tomato are softened, and then serve on romaine lettuce shells with toppings of your choice.

Spinach Salad

Servings 2
1 bag Baby Spinach
½ Red Pepper, diced
¼ Yellow Pepper, diced
½ cup Almonds, sliced
1 cup Broccoli, chopped
1 Avocado, peeled and diced
¼ cup Olive Oil
¼ cup Balsamic Vinegar
1 tsp. Garlic Powder
2 tsp. Black Pepper

Combine your olive oil and balsamic vinegar together to make a vinaigrette dressing. Add garlic powder and pepper to your dressing and mix. Next, combine all of your ingredients and toss them gently in your dressing.

Side Dishes

Green Beans and Almonds

Servings 4
4 Cups Fresh Green Beans
¼ Cup Diced Almonds
2 Cloves Garlic, minced
Salt and Pepper
Olive Oil

Place your diced almonds into a sauté pan and cook them for a few minutes in a little bit of olive oil. Add your fresh green beans, salt, pepper and garlic cloves and sauté until your green beans are bright green and still slightly crunchy.

Roasted Tomatoes and Squash

Servings 4
2 Large Tomatoes, sliced thinly
1 Large Zucchini, sliced thinly
1 Medium Squash, sliced thinly
2 tbsp. Olive Oil
3 Cloves Garlic, minced
½ tbsp. Black Pepper
½ tbsp. Salt

Line your tomatoes, zucchini and squash slices in a baking pan. Drizzle olive oil over them and sprinkle the veggies with garlic, salt and pepper. Bake in a 350 degree oven for 25-30 minutes.

Stuffed Baby Portobello Mushrooms

Servings 4
8 Baby Portobello Mushrooms, cleaned and de-stemmed
1 ½ Cup Spinach Leaves, chopped
½ Cup Tomato, diced
½ Cup Yellow Pepper, diced
1 Cup Brown Rice, cooked
Salt and Pepper to Taste
2 Cloves Garlic, minced
1 tbsp. Olive Oil

Clean and de-stem your baby Portobello mushrooms and chop the stems up finely. Add the stems to your cooked brown rice and then add tomato, garlic and yellow pepper. Next, sauté your spinach and add it to your rice mixture. Scoop the rice and veggie mixture into each mushroom and then bake for 20 minutes in the oven at 400 degrees.

Kale

Servings 4
1 Large Bunch of Kale, washed and chopped roughly
3 Cloves Garlic, minced
Salt and Pepper
Olive Oil

Sautee your minced garlic in olive oil for 2-3 minutes, and then add your kale, salt and pepper to the pan. Sautee for 3-5 minutes.

Vegetable and Egg Cups

Servings 6
12 Large Eggs
½ Cup Onion, diced
½ Cup Tomato, diced
½ Cup Broccoli, diced
¼ Cup Spinach Leaves, diced
½ tbsp. Garlic Salt
Salt and Pepper to Taste
Olive Oil

Drizzle olive oil in the bottom of a muffin tin. Then, mix your eggs, veggies and spices together until the egg yolks and whites have been incorporated. Pour your mixture evenly into the muffin tins and bake at 350 degrees for 10-15 minutes.

Garlic-Herb Sweet Potatoes

Servings 4
4 White Sweet Potatoes, diced
3 Cloves Garlic, minced
1 tbsp. Dried Basil
1 tbsp. Dried Oregano
½ tbsp. Black Pepper
2 tsp. Salt
2 tbsp. Olive Oil

Mix your potatoes in a bowl with olive oil and your spices. Sauté your garlic in a saucepan for 2-3 minutes then add the garlic to your potato mixture and then pour your potatoes into a baking pan and bake for 35-40 minutes at 375 degrees.

Quinoa and Vegetables

Servings 4
1 cup Quinoa
2 cups Vegetable Broth
1 Large Carrot, peeled and diced
3 Stalks Celery, diced
2 cups Cauliflower, chopped
1 tbsp. Black Pepper
3 Cloves Garlic, minced

Throw all of your ingredients into a soup pot and cook on high until the vegetable broth boils. Then, cover the mixture and simmer for the next 20 minutes. Add extra broth or water if the dish is dry.

Cauliflower Mash

Servings 4
1 Head Cauliflower, chopped roughly
1 tbsp. Olive Oil
1 tbsp. Basil
1 tbsp. Oregano
1 tbsp. Garlic Salt
½ tbsp. Onion Powder
Black Pepper to Taste
Water as Needed

Steam your cauliflower on the stove, or in the microwave then mash it with a fork. Add your olive oil and spices and continue to mash until the cauliflower becomes creamy. Add water as needed to help the cauliflower mash.

Asparagus and Bacon

Serves 4
1 lb. Asparagus, washed
1 lb. Bacon
Olive Oil
Salt and Pepper to Taste

Cook your bacon for 2 minutes on each side over medium heat in a frying pan. Then, drizzle olive oil on a baking sheet and lay your asparagus on the baking sheet. Sprinkle salt and pepper on the asparagus and then gently wrap each asparagus stalk with one piece of bacon. If you have extra bacon, wrap some of the asparagus with two strips of bacon. Place in your oven and cook on 350 until the bacon is crispy, usually around 20 minutes.

Brussels Sprouts

Serves 4
1 lb. Brussels Sprouts, cut in chunks
2 cloves Garlic, minced
1 tbsp. Olive Oil
1 tbsp. Onion Powder
Salt and Pepper to Taste
2 tbsp. Honey

Sauté your Brussels sprouts in 1 tbsp olive oil with the garlic, onion powder and salt and pepper. Cover the pan for 2 minutes and allow the veggies to steam on medium heat. Next, pour two tablespoons of honey over your Brussels sprouts and stir them in the sauté pan so that each piece of vegetable gets a bit of honey. Serve piping hot.

Roasted Peppers

Serves 4
1 Red Pepper, sliced
1 Yellow Pepper, sliced
2 cloves Garlic, minced
1 tbsp. Olive Oil
1 tsp. Onion Powder
Balsamic Vinegar
Salt and Pepper to Taste

Sauté the pepper slices in garlic and olive oil. Sprinkle the onion powder, salt and pepper onto the peppers and cook for 3-5 minutes until the peppers are still crunchy. Sprinkle with balsamic vinegar and oil to finish.

Sweet Corn

Serves 4
4 Sweet Corn Cobs, corn cut off
2 tbsp. Grass Fed Butter
2 cloves Garlic
2 tsp. Black Pepper
1 tsp. Salt
2 tsp. Paprika
¼ cup Onion, diced

Put the grass fed natural butter into a skillet and melt over medium heat. Next, pour the rest of your ingredients into the skillet and stir. Cook uncovered over medium heat for 10 minutes, stirring every few minutes.

Brown Rice Salad

Serves 4
2 Large Carrots, peeled and diced
½ cup Cucumber, diced
½ cup Celery, diced
5 Small Radishes, sliced
1 cup Peas
3 cups Brown Rice
2 tbsp. Honey
2 tbsp. Olive Oil
½ tsp. Salt
½ tsp. Black Pepper
5 Basil Leaves, roughly chopped
5 Parsley Leaves, roughly chopped

Combine all of the ingredients in a large bowl and mix thoroughly. Make sure that your brown rice is cooled completely before you add it to the salad. Chill the salad for 2 hours in the refrigerator and serve cold.

Zucchini Noodles

Serves 4
2 Large Zucchini, sliced thinly
2 tbsp. Olive Oil
¼ cup Fresh Basil
1 tsp. Salt
2 tsp. Black Pepper

Cut your zucchini thin by using a mandolin in order to form zucchini ribbons. Next, boil the zucchini ribbons in salted water until they are tender. Once cooked, drain the zucchini ribbons and toss in basil, olive oil and pepper. Serve hot.

Broccoli with Garlic

Serves 4
1 Head of Broccoli, chopped
2 cloves Garlic, minced
1 tbsp. Olive Oil
1 tbsp. Lemon Juice
½ tsp. Red Pepper Flakes
Salt and Pepper to Taste

Sauté your broccoli and garlic in a skillet with olive oil. Once the broccoli is bright green and still crunchy remove from the heat and add the lemon juice, red better flakes, salt and pepper. Stir the broccoli in the mixture and then serve.

Rainbow Chard with Shiitake Mushrooms

Serves 4
1 Large Bunch of Rainbow Chard
½ lb. Shiitake Mushrooms, cleaned
1 tbsp. Grass Fed Natural Butter
3 cloves Garlic, minced
½ cup White Onion, diced
½ cup Water
Salt and Pepper to Taste

Cut the stems off of your rainbow chard and discard. Then, cut the leaves off of the chard and separate the remaining stems and leaves. Cut the stems into 1 inch pieces and add them to a skillet with your butter, onion and mushrooms. Cook over medium heat until the stems have softened. Then add your garlic, and a pinch of salt and pepper. Next, add the chard leaves and cook until they have wilted completely. Add your water and cover the pan. Simmer for 3-5 minutes, or until all of the rainbow chard leaves have wilted. Serve hot, and re-season with salt and pepper if needed.

Desserts

Fruity Popsicles

Servings 6
3 Bananas
½ cup Strawberries
½ cup Blueberries
1 cup Spinach
½ cup Coconut Milk

Throw all of your ingredients into a high powdered blender and blend until smooth. Then, pour your mixture into a popsicle mold and place them into the freezer. Freeze the popsicles overnight and then enjoy.

Paleo Pancakes and Fruit

Servings 6
6 Ripe Bananas
3 Large Eggs
1 tsp. Cinnamon
1 tsp. Nutmeg
1 tbsp. Honey
Strawberries and Blueberries for Toppings

Mash up the bananas until they are smooth, then add the eggs and beat thoroughly. Next, add the cinnamon, nutmeg and honey to the mixture and stir. To cook, pour the mixture into a hot skillet and cook each pancake for 2-3 minutes per side. Top your finished pancakes with strawberries and blueberries, or any type of seasonal fruit and enjoy.

Banana Bread

Servings 6
5 Ripe Bananas
4 Large Eggs
½ cup Peanut Butter
4 tbsp. Coconut Oil
½ cup Rice Flour
1 tbsp. Cinnamon
1 tsp. Baking Soda
1 tsp. Vanilla
1 tsp. Baking Powder
3 tsp. Nutmeg

Combine 4 of the bananas, the eggs and the peanut butter together and mix thoroughly. Mash your bananas until they reach a liquid consistency. Next, add the coconut oil and blend the mixture with a hand mixer. Next, add the rice flour, baking soda, baking powder, and your spices. Pour the mixture into a bread pan, and cut up your last banana and sprinkle it on top of the bread pan. Bake the bread at 350 degrees for 60 minutes.

Mixed Berry Rice

Servings 6
2 cups Brown Rice, Cooked
1 cup Blueberries
2 tbsp. Honey
1 cup Strawberries, diced
½ tbsp. Cinnamon
½ cup Coconut Milk

Add your cooked rice to a saucepan with the coconut milk. Allow the rice to heat up over medium heat. Next, add your strawberries and blueberries and simmer until the fruit has been broken down slightly. Next, add the cinnamon and honey and stir. Allow the mixture to cook for 10 minutes on low and then serve piping hot. Add extra coconut milk for extra creaminess if desired.

Banana Bread Truffles

Servings 6
Paleo Banana Bread (see recipe on pg. 19)
1 cup Water
1/3 cup Cocoa
½ cup Maple Syrup

Combine the water, cocoa and maple syrup in a saucepan and stir until the cocoa powder has been incorporated. Simmer the mixture for 10 minutes while you stir briskly. Next, grab your already made banana bread and while the chocolate sauce is cooling, crumble it into little pieces. Next, form small balls out of the banana bread crumbles by rolling the bread in your hands like dough. Then, dip the bread balls into the chocolate sauce and place them on a baking
sheet to cool. The chocolate sauce should harden and you will be left with chocolate covered banana bread bites. Sprinkle the bites with extra cinnamon or honey if desired.

Paleo Pie Crust

Servings 8
1 ½ cup Sweet Rice Flour
½ cup Almonds
¼ cup Coconut Oil
¼ cup Honey
1 tsp. Vanilla

Place all of the ingredients into a food processor and blend. The blended mixture should appear dough-like. If it doesn't, then add extra coconut oil to keep the dry crumbles together. If the dough is too wet, then add extra almonds or sweet rice flour. Next, place the dough into a pie pan and spread it evenly into the pan. Place the crust in the freezer for 3 hours and then add your favorite filling and serve.

Blueberry Pie Filling

Servings 8
5 cups Fresh or Frozen Blueberries
1/8 cup Honey
¼ cup Arrowroot Starch
½ tsp Salt

Mix the ingredients together and then pour them into a saucepan and cook on low for 10-15 minutes while stirring constantly. Next, pour the ingredients into the prepared pie crust (pg. 20) and chill the pie. Serve cold after it has been chilled in the refrigerator for 2 hours.

Strawberry Banana Pie Filling

Servings 6
3 Ripe Bananas
2 Cups Strawberries, sliced
1 tbsp. Fresh Lemon Juice
1/3 cup Coconut Milk
1/8 cup Honey

Mash the bananas and add the lemon juice, coconut milk and honey. Layer this mixture into a pre-made pie crust (pg. 20) and then layer sliced strawberries on top of the banana mixture. Place the pie in the refrigerator for 2 hours to chill. Then serve cold.

Strawberry Pie Filling

Servings 8
5 cups Fresh or Frozen Strawberries, diced
1/8 cup Honey
¼ cup Arrowroot Starch
½ tsp Salt

Mix the ingredients together and then pour them into a saucepan and cook on low for 10-15 minutes while stirring constantly. Next, pour the ingredients into the prepared pie crust (pg. 20) and chill the pie. Serve cold after it has been chilled in the refrigerator for at least two hours. It is best if chilled overnight.

Rice Balls

Servings 10
3 cups White Rice, cooked
½ cup Coconut Milk
¼ cup Coconut Oil
2 cups Blueberries
½ cup Honey

Place the blueberries, coconut milk and coconut oil into a saucepan and simmer for 10 minutes while stirring. Then, add the rice and the honey to the mixture and stir. Cook for another 10 minutes, and then remove from the heat and allow the mixture to cool and thicken. Once the mixture is cooled and has thickened, scoop out one tablespoon servings of the mixture and roll them into balls. Then, place them on a baking sheet and place the baking sheet in the refrigerator overnight for them to set. If your rice mixture never thickens, then add a little bit of arrowroot starch or tapioca starch to help the process along. Start with 1 tbsp and then go up from there.

Banana Boats

Servings 8
8 Bananas, cut in half lengthwise
½ cup Almond Butter
¼ cup Raisins
¼ cup Almonds
¼ cup Carob Chips
¼ cup Strawberries, diced finely
Lemon Juice

Lay each of your bananas on a foil lined baking sheet. Brush the bananas with lemon juice to keep them from turning brown. Next, spread almond butter onto each banana and then begin adding your other ingredients to each banana half. Once all of the ingredients have been added, tent the baking sheet with foil and place it in the freezer overnight.